I0488082

A Peep into Medical Antiquity

A Peep into Medical Antiquity

By
N. H. Kassabian, M.D.
Edited by Chris Heimler

iUniverse, Inc.
New York Lincoln Shanghai

A Peep into Medical Antiquity

All Rights Reserved © 2004 by Chris Heimler

No part of this book may be reproduced or transmitted in any form or by any means, graphic, electronic, or mechanical, including photocopying, recording, taping, or by any information storage retrieval system, without the written permission of the publisher.

iUniverse, Inc.

For information address:
iUniverse, Inc.
2021 Pine Lake Road, Suite 100
Lincoln, NE 68512
www.iuniverse.com

Front cover art courtesy of Walter "Paul" G. Brand IV.

ISBN: 0-595-33501-2

Printed in the United States of America

This book is dedicated to the Armenian people and all they have done for the world. Although they have undergone many hardships and trials as a people, the Armenians have retained their dignity, humanity, and compassion. They are a driving force in the world today and continue to raise up extraordinary persons from their ranks. May they continue as they have until now and be blessed for all they have done thus far. A portion of the proceeds for this book will go to aid the Armenian National Science & Education Fund. You can visit their website and find out more about this upstanding organization by going to http://www.ansef.org.

"Out of the heterogeneous elements the new American race will come, supreme in arts, sciences, culture, and civilization, and we Armenians shall be proud to think that we, as a racial element, have contributed our share into the creation and development of this new race."

—N. H. Kassabian

CONTENTS

▼

Foreword

My research on the late Dr. Nushan H. Kassabian began in 1997, soon after I discovered the doctor lived and practiced medicine in my home for 26 years. I was able to contact a relative of Dr. Kassabian who lived nearby and obtained many of the doctor's medical instruments, photos, pamphlets and medical books, some of the latter dating back to the 1890's. While going through the pamphlets, I came upon a speech he had read before the Ottawa and Kent County Medical Societies. It was entitled, "A Peep Into Medical Antiquity." After reading the doctor's words, I felt sure this pamphlet should be printed and shared with universities across America.

"A Peep Into Medical Antiquity" is a glimpse into the history of medicine and those who founded many of the practices we use today. Dr. Kassabian expresses his own views on the history of medicine and how ancient cultures practiced. You will also read how ancient ways differed from current practices as well as many similarities.

Dr. Kassabian, physician and surgeon, always believed that anyone in the medical profession should dedicate themselves entirely to their work and this, I believe, is what made the doctor different from many physicians of his day.

After his wife, Margerite's, death in 1911, he dedicated his entire life to medicine and many remember him working around the clock in his Detroit laboratory.

Acknowledgments

I would like to thank: The Kassabian Family, David Van Koevering & Family, The New York Public Library, and Ruth Z. Lewis for her help on research, the Heimler family, Mr. and Mrs. James Dahnke and family, the Burgenmeyer family, John Perrin, my Grandmother Alice E. Perrin, my mother Susan M. Slattery, Central Michigan University, Northwestern University in Chicago, Detroit Public Library, Highland Park Public Library (Detroit), Former Secretary of the Navy Paul R. Ignatius, Perry McClellen, Grand Rapids Public Library, *The Grand Rapids Press* (various editions). Northeast Ottawa District Library (Coopersville, MI), *Detroit Free Press, Ottawa Advance* Newspapers, *The Coopersville Observer* 1880–1975, *Coopersville Observer* 1995 to present, Jeff Parish and family, Morris Parrish and family, Michigan Medical Society, the citizens of Detroit for their help and encouragement, Glendale Public Library (California), Los Angeles Public Library, The citizens of Grand Rapids for their help and support, Michigan State Archives, the citizens of Coopersville, MI for their help and support, Ross Conran for encouragement, Ron Veldman for help and encouragement, the City Government of Coopersville, Michigan Department of Health, Richard Cryderman and family for believing in me, Grand Haven Court House, Robert A. Kuiper—Creative Photography Inc., University of Michigan—Bentley Library,.

I owe special thanks to: Mr. and Mrs. Craig A. Hart, Paul Brand, Craig S. Boyer for telling me to never quit. Professor Mrs. Lynne Wood (Muskegon Community College), Dr. Joe Van Koevering and family for preaching the word of God to me (over the phone), the Armenian National Science and Education Fund and the Fund for Armenian Relief for all their support, and a very special thanks to the Lord above for helping me reach my dreams.

A Peep Into Medical Antiquity

The history of medicine, its origin, in the dim of antiquity, and its development, has an intimate connection with the progress of philosophy, religion and science, in other words, civilization at large. Medicine, being an art even during the embryonic stage of its existence, grew parallel with its sister fine arts. Where did medicine originate? Where was its cradle? Shall we unhesitatingly and with an implicit confidence believe, as some of the ancient writers did, that Athens, the classic city of the Hellenic race, was the mother of arts, as Milton is pleased to call her? Now for a moment I wish to become an insurgent. It seems to be very much *a la mode* nowadays, and I wish to claim that Milton and the rest of his followers are very much mistaken. Milton is unquestionably an authority on Paradise Lost. He makes, however, a gross mistake when, in his great admiration of Grecian culture, he says: "O Athens, Mother of Arts." The prevailing opinion was those days that Athens was the originator and propagator of Arts. Kurt Sprengel, in his "Histoire de la Medicine," says: "Greece, this favored spot of Nature, was of all others the fittest for the birthplace of medicine and other sciences and arts." (1815) But the fact is that the pick and shovel of Layard in Nineveh and recent excavations have made some marvelous revelations in regard to the origin of art in general. We have been compelled by an over-whelming majority of facts and an abundance of material to admit that in order to find the cradle of arts we need not linger round the Athenian acropolis. We ought to make a pilgrimage to the banks of the Nile and the Euphrates, because on the shores of these most ancient rivers, art originated, was nursed to maturity and from there transmitted, if I may express myself in this manner, to Asia Minor and Greece. We must admit that the Greek genius gave to it an impetus, improving the art which they had learned from the Egyptians, Phœnicians and Assyrians and, in due course of time, imparting it to the Romans and to the world.

Men during this early period of existence, while believing a polytheistic religion, in their fancy attributed all forms of sickness, mental or bodily suffering, to the displeasure of some one of their deities and, of course, to such deities turn with petitions, prayers and sacrifices for relief. A large majority of the people of the Orient still believe that for fever they have to appeal to a certain saint, for safe travel to some other, for sterility to still another one with sacrificial offerings, thus proving that even after the introduction of Christianity, old pagan ideas had still their sway in the minds of the people.

Among the nations of remote antiquity that attained a higher and enviable level in the cultivation of arts, Egypt stood as the one *par excellence.* Marpero, one of the most renowned Egyptologists of this century, estimates the beginning of the Egyptian civilization somewhere between six and seven thousand years before Christ.

In Egypt, as well as among the nations of southwestern Asia, the universal belief was that both diseases and their remedies were derived from and controlled by their deities, necessarily caused the office of priest and physician to be united in the same person, and the temples for worship became the chief places of resort for the sick. The most noted of Egyptian temples were at Thebes, Memphis and Heliopolis.

It is perhaps interesting to mention the names of four physicians who are represented as practicing medicine between 5000 to 4000 B. C.—Teta, Tsethosta, Nebsu and Chai. The first two were also kings, and the last was an occultist.

"If I wished to characterize in one word," says Schlegel, "the peculiar bearing and ruling element of the Egyptian mind—however un-satisfactory in other respects such general designation may be—I should say that the intellectual eminence of that people was in its scientific profundity—in an understanding that penetrated, or sought to penetrate, by magic, into all the depths and mysteries of Nature; even into their most hidden abyss. So thoroughly scientific was the whole learning and character of the Egyptian mind that even the architecture of this people had an astronomical import, even far more than that of the other nations of early antiquity. I have already had occasion to speak of their treatment of the dead. In all the natural sciences, in mathematics, astronomy, and even in medicine, they were the masters of the Greeks; and even the profoundest thinkers among the latter, the Pythagoreans, and afterwards the great Plato himself, derived from them the first elements of their doctrines, or caught at least the first outline of the mighty speculations. Here, too, in the birth place of hieroglyphics, was the chief seat of the mysteries, and Egypt has at all times been the native country of many true, as well as many false, secrets."

Every month the Egyptians, according to Maspero, for three successive days, purged the system by means of emetics or clysters. The study of medicine with them was divided between specialists, each physician attending to one kind of illness only. Every place possessed several doctors, some for the diseases, the bone setters attached to the worship of Sakhit, who treated fractures by the intercession of the goddess, and the exorcist who professed to cure by the sole virtue of amulets and magic phrases. The professional doctor treated all kinds of maladies, but as with us, there were specialists for certain affections who were consulted in preference to general practitioners.

The climatic character of the country necessitated the presence of a considerable number of specialists. Where ophthalmia and affections of the intestines predominated, we necessarily find many occultists, as well as doctors for internal maladies. The best instructed, however, knew but little of anatomy. As with the Christian physicians of the Middle Ages, religious scruples prevented the Egyptians from cutting or dissecting in the cause of pure science the dead body which was identified with that of Osiris. The processes of embalming, which would have instructed them in anatomy, were not entrusted to doctors. The knowledge of what went on within the body was therefore but vague. Life seemed to be a little air, a breath which was conveyed by veins from member to member. Under the influence of the good breaths, the vessels were inflated and worked regularly, under that of the evil they became inflamed, were obstructed, were hardened, or gave away and the physician had to remove the obstruction, allay the inflammation, and reestablish their vigor and elasticity. At the moment of death the vital spirits withdrew with the soul, the blood deprived of air "became coagulated, the veins and arteries emptied themselves and the creature perished for want of breath."

The majority of diseases from which the ancient Egyptians suffered are those which still attack their successors: ophthalmia, affections of the stomach, abdomen and bladder, intestinal parasites, varicose veins, ulcers in the leg, the Nile pimples and finally the divine mortal malady, the *divinus morbus* of the Latins, epilepsy. Anemia, from which at least one-fourth of the present population suffers, was not less prevalent than at present, if we may judge from the number of remedies, which were used against hematuria, the principal cause of it.

Egyptian physicians were able, however, to determine fairly well specific characteristics of ordinary affections and sometimes describe them in a precise and graphic fashion. "The abdomen is heavy, the pit of the stomach painful, the heart burns and palpitates violently. The clothing oppresses the sick man and he can hardly support it, nocturnal thirsts. His heart is sick as that of a man who has eaten of the sycamore gum." This is the beginning of gastric fevers so common in Egypt. A modern physician could not better diagnose such a case; the phraseology would be less flowery but the analysis of the symptoms would not differ from that given us by the ancient practitioner of remote antiquity.

The medicaments recommended comprise nearly everything, which can in some way or other be swallowed, whether in solid, mucilaginous or liquid form. Vegetable remedies are reckoned by the score, from the most modest herb to the largest tree, such as sycamore, palm, acacia and cedar, of which the sawdust and shavings were supposed to posses both antiseptic and emollient properties. Among the mineral substances are to be noted sea salt, alum, niter, sulphate of copper, and a score of different kinds of stones; among the latter the Memphite stone was distinguished for its virtue—if applied to the parts of the body which were lacerated or unhealthy it acted as an anesthetic and facilitated the success of surgical operations.

The medicaments compounded of these incongruous substances were often very complicated. It was thought that multiplying the curative elements increased the healing power; each ingredient acted on a specific region of the body. The physician made use of all the means we employ today to introduce remedies into the human system, whether pills or potions, poultices or ointments, draughts or clysters. Not only did he give the prescriptions, but he made them up, thus combining the art of physician with that of a dispenser. He prescribed the ingredients, pounded them either separately or together, he macerated them in the proper way, boiled them, reduced them by heating, and filtered through linen. Fat served him as the ordinary vehicle for ointments and pure water for potions; but he did not despise other liquids, such as wine, beer, vinegar, milk, olive oil, even the urine of men and animals; the whole sweetened with honey was taken hot night and morning. The use of more than one of these remedies became worldwide. The Greeks borrowed them from the Egyptians; we have piously accepted them from the Greeks; and our contemporaries still swallow with resignation many of the abominable mixtures invented on the banks of the Nile and Euphrates in the dim of remote antiquity long before the building of the pyramids.

Chaldea abounded with soothsayers and necromancers no less than with astrologers; she possessed no real school of medicine, such as we find in Egypt, in which were taught rational methods of diagnosing maladies and of curing them by the use remedies. The Chaldeans are content to confide the care of their bodies to sorcerers and exorcists who were experts in the art of casting out demons and spirits whose presence in a living being brought about those disorders to which humanity is prone.

The facial expression of the patient during the crisis, the words which escaped from him delirium, were, for these clever individuals, so many signs revealing the nature and sometimes the name of the enemy to be combated, the fear-god, the plague-god, the headache-god.

Consultations and medical treatment were, therefore, religious offices, in which were involved purifications, offerings and a whole ritual of mysterious words and gestures. The magician lighted a fire of herbs and sweet smelling plants in front of his patient, and the clear flame rising from this put the specters to flight and dispelled the malign influence.

The medical authorities in Chaldea recommended such remedies, which were for the most part both grotesque and disgusting in their composition. They comprised bitter and stinking wood shaving, raw meat, Soakis flesh, wine and oil, the whole reduced to a pulp or made into a sort of pill and swallowed. They attributed to these compounds wonderful effects, these strange compositions were recommended before all others, and their very strangeness reassured the patient as to their efficacy.

The Chaldeans were not, however, ignorant of the natural virtues of herbs and at times made use of them; but they were not held in very high esteem, and the physicians preferred the prescriptions, which pandered to the popular craving for the supernatural.

Amulets further confirmed the effect produced by the recipes, and prevented the enemy, once cast out, from reentering the body; these amulets were made of knots of cord, pierced shell, bronze or terra cotta statuettes and plaques fastened to the arms or worn around the neck. On each of the latter kind were roughly drawn the most terrible images that they could conceive, a shortened incantation was scrawled on its surface, or it was covered with extraordinary characters, which, when the spirits perceived, they at once took flight and the possessor of the talisman escaped the threatened illness.

The following is a specimen of an Assyrian physician's writing to the King:

"To the king, my lord, thy servant, Arad Nana, Greeting most heartily to my Lord, the King. May Adar and Gala grant health of mind and body to my Lord, the King. A Hearty greeting to the Son of the King.

"With regard to the patient who has a bleeding from his nose, the Rab-Magi reports: 'Yesterday, towards evening, there was much hemorrhage.' These dressings are not scientifically applied. They are placed on the alae of the nose, oppress the breathing and come off when there is hemorrhage. Let them be placed within the nostrils and then the air will be kept away and the hemorrhage restrained. If it is agreeable to my Lord, the King, I will go to-morrow and give instructions, meantime let me hear how he does."

*Another specimen of Assyrian
Correspondence:*

"To the King My Lord, thy servant Arad Nana, may thereby place forever and ever to the King my Lord. May the God Nina and the Goddess Gula give soundness of heart and soundness of flesh to the King my Lord, peace forever.

"To reduce the general inflammation of his forehead, I have tied a bandage upon it. His face is swollen; yesterday as formerly, I opened the wound, which had been received in the midst of it. As for the bandage which was over the swelling, matter was upon the bandage, the size of the tip of the little finger."

They have also another institution, says Herodotus, the good tendency of which claims applause. Such as are diseased among them they carry into some public square. They have no professors of medicine, but the passengers in general interrogate the sick person concerning his malady, that if any person has either been afflicted with a similar disease himself, or seen its operation on another, he may communicate the process by which his own recovery was affected, or by which in any other instance he knew the disease to be removed. No one may pass by the affected person in silence or without inquiry into the nature of his complaint.

ASSYRIAN PRESCRIPTION FOR THE DISEASE OF THE HEAD BY CAMPBELL THOMPSON

"When a man's brain contains fire and myalgia afflicts the temples and smites the eye so that his eyes are affected with dimness, cloudiness, a disturbed appearance with the veins bloodshot, shedding tears, pound one-third of a Ka of Shila with a pestle until thou hast strained it; add one-third of a ka of Sak-Ka-a-kal thereto and knead it in an infusion of cassia, press, bind it on (as a poultice) and do not take it off for three days."

FROM THE MOST ANCIENT CODE RELATIVE TO THE PRACTICE OF MEDICINE

From the code of Khammurabi:

"If a doctor has treated a man for severe wound with a lancet of bronze and has cured the man or has opened a tumor with a bronzed lancet and has cured the man's eye he shall receive ten shekels of silver.

"If a physician has treated a free borne man for a severe wound with a lancet of bronze and has caused the man to die, or has opened a tumor of the man with a lancet of bronze and has destroyed his eye, his hands shall be cut off.

"If a doctor has treated the slave of a freed man for a severe wound with a bronzed lancet and has caused him to die he shall give back slave for slave. If he has opened his tumor with a bronzed lancet and has ruined his eye he shall pay the half of his price in money.

"If a doctor has cured the broken limb of a man or has healed his sick body the patient shall pay the doctor five shekels of silver.

"If a doctor of oxen and asses has treated an ox or an ass for a grave wound and has cured it the owner of the ox or ass shall give to the doctor as his pay one-sixth of a shekel of silver. If he has treated an ox or an ass for a severe wound and has caused its death he shall pay one-fourth of its price to the owner of the ox or ass."

There is no nation in southwestern Asia to which modern civilization and culture is as much indebted as the Israelitic race, and still so little appreciated, and more than that often submitted to disdain, ridicule and persecution. This being the case, I will take a few moments to show the impress of Hebraic civilization.

Our present mode of thought and feeling, our lives and actions are far more profoundly influenced by the world of thought and feeling which Israel created, than by that of Greece or Rome. Our whole civilization today is saturated and permeated with tendencies and impulses, which have their origin in Judea. The reason for this is that in Israel one side of human nature had developed to very great perfection, a side which is of far greater consequence to mankind in general than art and science, law or philosophy. While in Hellas, philosophy first, and then indirectly science developed out of mythology, in Israel the age of mythology was succeeded by that of religion; and we may say that the religion of Israel is still the active religion of mankind, as maintained by Bernard Stade, in a far higher degree than the philosophy of the Greeks is still its active philosophy. What Israel did in the sphere of religion is without a doubt far more epoch-making, unique and effective than what the Romans did in the sphere of politics or the Greeks in that of art and science.

It was the strong belief of the Jews that disease and especially epidemics were sent as punishments by the deities on account of their sins. Consequently, for relief, they resorted to repentance, prayer and the interposition of the priests officiating in their places of worship, rather than to the administration of medicines. They thereby combined the function of priest and physician in the same persons. Moses, their great lawgiver, gave them the earliest elementary code of public hygiene of which we have any record. It contained specific directions of food; the slaughtering of animals; the burial of the dead; the regulation of marriage and sexual relations; the diagnosis and isolation of cases of leprosy and the strict prohibition of artificial abortion.

It is clear that Homer attributes such superiority to several eastern nations, more especially to the Phœnicians, not only in wealth, but in knowledge and skill, that compared with their progress, the arts of Greece seem to be in their infancy. The description of a Phœnician vessel, which comes to a Greek island freighted with trinkets, and of the manner in which a lady of the highest rank, and her servants, handle and gaze on one of the foreign ornaments, presents the image of such commerce as Europeans carry on with the islanders of the South Sea now.

The chances of war give occasion, as might be expected, for frequent allusions to the healing art. The Greek Army contains two chiefs who have inherited consummate skill in this art from their father, Æsculapius; and Achilles has been so well instructed in it by Chiron that Patroclus, to whom he has imparted his knowledge, is able to supply their place. The operation of extracting a weapon from the wound with a knife seems not to have been considered as one, which demanded peculiar skill; the science of the physician was chiefly displayed in the application of medicinal herbs, by which he stanched the blood and eased the pain. When Ulysses has been gored by a wild boar his friends first bind up the hurt and then use a charm for stopping the flow of blood. The healing art, such as it was, was frequently and successfully practiced by the women.

The fifth century B. C. was a period when Greek civilization and power had reached their zenith. Greece had victoriously closed her wars with Persia, and in statesmanship, in works of art, in history, in schools of philosophy and in physical culture she had excelled all her contemporaries. The art of writing had been introduced from Phœnicia and the use of papyrus from Egypt, thereby greatly facilitating the recording of facts and the history of events of every kind. It was at this auspicious period in human progress that Hippocrates, justly surnamed the "Father of Medical Literature" as well as the "Father of Medicine," was born on the Island of Cos, about 460 B. C. His father, Heraclides, belonged to the order of Æsclepiadæ. Hippocrates received his early education under his parents in the Temple. He went to Athens where he was educated in the best schools of Greece, and thoroughly acquainted with whatever records relating to medical topics had accumulated in the Æsclepion at Cos, which was one of the most celebrated then in existence. He commenced his professional career contemporaneous with the statesmen Themistocles, Miltiades, Pericles and Nicias; the philosophers Anaxagoras, Pythagoras, Socrates and Plato; the dramatists Æschylus, Sophocles, and Eurypides; the orators Lysias and Demosthenes; and the historians Thucydides, Herodotus and Xenophon.

Hippocrates was the first to separate himself from the order of Æsclepiadæ in which he had been born, and engaged in the work of a general practitioner of medicine. As such he visited and practiced in the provinces of Thessaly, Macedonia and Scythia, and everywhere he studied with great care the actual phenomena of diseases and their etiology. He died in Larissa, Thessaly, in about 377 B. C. His reputation is said to have greatly increased by his successful treatment and cure of Perdicas, king of Macedonia, who was sorely afflicted with love sickness.

One of the characteristic precepts of Hippocrates is worthy of the attention of every practitioner of medicine, and I quote it as follows:

"Life is short, opportunity fleeting, judgment difficult, treatment easy, thought hard; but treatment after thought is proper and profitable."

Equally worthy of remembrance are the following maxims: "The physician is a servant, not a teacher, of Nature. Follow Nature." The physician should benefit, or at least not injure; yet he declares that, "timidity indicates incapacity, rashness want of skill." We might say that the three distinguishing mental qualities of Hippocrates were patient observation, logical reasoning and faithful recording of both facts and deductions.

A much more important practitioner and contributor to medical literature was Soronnes of Ephesus, who practiced in Rome during the time of Trajan and Hadrian, from 98 A. D. to 138 A. D. His works on midwifery show that practical obstetrics was at that time relatively better understood than any other branch of medicine.

Claudius Galen, the most important man Asia Minor has produced in the field of medicine, after Hippocrates, was born at Pergamus, 131 A. D. At the age of 15, he commenced the study of the prevailing systems of philosophy and of medicine, first at Pergamus and later at Corinth. At the age of 21, he went to Smyrna and visited most of the interesting places in Asia Minor and Palestine. He went to Alexandria and spent considerable time in the great library and museum, and was much interested in the study of the complete human skeleton contained in the museum.

At the age of 28 he returned to his native city, Pergamus, and engaged in the practice of medicine in connection with the gymnasium, and rapidly acquired a high reputation. Six years later, he changed his residence to Rome, where he not only engaged in general practice but also in lecturing on anatomy and physiology, and by his unusual attainments and industry he soon attracted general attention. He went back to Pergamus but one year later he was induced by the emperor, Marcus Aurelius, to again visit Rome, where he became physician in ordinary to the ruler and continued there until the end of his life, about 206 A. D. He was a very industrious student and prolific writer on a wide range of subjects. His works on grammatical, mathematical, philosophical and legal subjects numbered 125. His independent works on medicine were eighty-three and his commentaries on the works of Hippocrates were fifteen. His treatises on medical subjects were called canonical because they remained the chief medical textbooks through the Middle Ages, or more than 1,000 years.

The old statement that there is nothing new under the sun seems again to be verified in the statement that Laennec, to whom is attributed the discovery of the method of physical diagnosis, inspection, palpation, percussion and auscultation, was not the originator of these methods, but only perfected their use as an art. Cordell (Bull. *Johns Hopkins Hosp., December, 1909*) calls attention to the fact that Aretæus, the Cappadocian, a successor to Hippocrates, a student of his works, and a contemporary of Galen in the second century of the Christian era practiced all these methods. Aretæus, as disclosed in his writings, was a very acute observer, and by inspection of his patients noted the character of the respiration, posture, decubitus, color, heat and swelling of the surface, the condition of the veins, tongue, pulse, nails, sputum, etc. He likewise resorted to palpation in enlargement of the liver and spleen, and notes the change in the position of ascitic fluid with change in posture of the patient, and by percussion noted tympanites, saying that the abdomen when tapped sounded like a drum. Hippocrates describes râles in diseases of the lungs, such as pneumonia, phthisis, empyema, etc., and they are referred to by Cælius Aurelianus in the fifth century A. D. and by Paul of Ægina in the seventh century. The term *percussion* is used by Aretæus in describing the symptoms of asthma, a name which evidently embraced other conditions giving rise to dyspnea, besides that to which we limit it. Hippocrates also laid much stress on succussion sounds in empyema. It is a fact of the highest interest that Aretæus recognized heart murmurs by auscultation, and he seems the only one of the ancient writers who auscultated the heart.

Constantine was the first of the Roman emperors to embrace the Christian religion, and in 312 A. D. proclaimed at Rome religious toleration. In 330, he moved his seat of government to Byzantium, which subsequently took the name of Constantinople. It was by decree of Emperor Constantine that the pagan institutions of Æsclepiadæ and all medical institutions under pagan control or Greco-Roman philosophy that recognized the worship of many gods were confiscated. The emperor's mother, Helena, at the same period was devoting much of her time and means to the founding of a general hospital for the sick and poor in Jerusalem. Another hospital was established at Antioch about 363 and still another noted one was organized at Cæsarea.

The Egyptians were the aristocrats of antiquity. It is true that the Greeks described all non-Hellenic nations as barbarians, but by no means did they regard all other nations as less civilized than themselves. To be sure, they did hold this attitude toward the Romans, Persians, Scythians and various other contemporary nations, but they made an exception in the case of the Egyptians. They regarded these people with something akin to reverence, as a people who could claim an antiquity of civilization to which Greece could not at all pretend.

It was gladly admitted by the Greeks that these oriental civilizations had flowered while Greek culture was yet in the bud. Solon, the lawgiver, was reported to have traveled in Egypt, and to have been widely patronized by the Egyptian priests as the representative of an infant race. An Egyptian priest lectured the famous Greek in this manner: "O Solon! Solon! You Hellenes are but children." Herodotus, though ostensibly writing of the Persian War, devoted whole sections of his history to Egypt, and accepts, as did his countrymen, the Egyptian claim to immense antiquity. Plato even resided for some years in Egypt, as Diodorus tells us, in the hope of gaining an insight into the mysteries of oriental philosophy. Nothing is more explicit than the testimony of Diodorus who, writing some three centuries after what we now speak of as the Golden Age of Greece, plainly indicates that not Greece, but Mesopotamia was looked to in his day as the classic land of culture, and we of today are enabled to catch glimpses of the data on which that estimate was based and to understand that fabled glory of ancient Assyria was no myth but a very tangible reality.

The history of Babylonia has an interest of wider kind than that of Egypt from its more intimate connections with the general history of the human race and from the remarkable influence, which its religion, its science and its civilizations have had on all subsequent human progress. Its religious traditions, carried away by the Israelites, who came out from the Ur of the Chaldeas (Genesis, xi, 31) have through this wonderful people become the heritage of all mankind; while its science and civilization through the medium of the Greeks and the Romans have become the basis of modern research and advancement.

Babylonian culture was the oldest in the world, and at the same time was the mother of all other civilizations of antiquity, as has been claimed by Hammel. It is possible that even the Egyptians derived some of the elements of their culture from the Babylonians or Chaldeans.

The world historic relations of Mesopotamian art are best brought out by a study of the later and more perfectly preserved examples of Assyrian craftsmanship. It was the Assyrian who borrowed more directly from the Babylonians and the Egyptians in developing his art and who passed those artistic impulses to the Persians on the one hand and the Greeks on the other. The monuments of Assyria furnish us with very important data as to the origin of many branches of art, subsequently brought to the highest perfection in Asia Minor and Greece. The indirect period of this influence is fully and completely illustrated by the monuments of Asia Minor of the time of Persian domination. The Zantian marbles acquired for England by Sir Charles Fellows and now in the British Museum are remarkable illustrations of the three-fold connection between Assyria and Persia, Persia and Asia Minor, and Asia Minor and Greece.

Were those marbles properly arranged and placed in chronological order, they would afford a most useful lesson and would enable even a superficial observer to trace the gradual progress of art from its primitive rudeness to the most classic conception of the Greek sculptor. Not that he would find either style the pure Assyrian or the Greek in its greatest perfection, but he would be able to see how a closer imitation of Nature, a gradual refinement of taste, an additional study had converted the hard and rigid lines of Assyrian into the following draperies and classic forms of the highest order or art. This second period has been termed that of indirect influence because the arts did not then penetrate directly into Asia Minor from Assyria, but were conveyed thither through the Persians. The Persians introduced into Asia Minor not only the arts but the religion as well that they received from the Assyrians. Thus, the tombs at Xantas and at Persepolis show a gradual progress in the mode of treatment, the introduction of action and sentiment and the knowledge of anatomy which mark the distinction between Asiatic and Greek art. Many architectural ornaments known to the Assyrians passed from them directly or indirectly into Greece. The Ionic column is an instance.

The three fundamental canons, "proportion, action and aspect," have been successfully met in all Assyrian art. The bas-relief of a wounded lion in a British Museum will prove this assertion. Still, though these bas-reliefs have an intrinsic worth as works of art their chief value is for what they teach regarding the evolution of art in the world. Before their discovery, it had been supposed that the stiff formalism of the Egyptian sculpture represented the fullest flight of the pre-Grecian art and that Greek art itself had stepped suddenly forth, rather a new creation than an evolution. But, as I said previously, the pick and shovel of Layard at Nineveh dispelled that illusion, for these art treasures that had lain there under the deposits of centuries were found to represent an enormous advance on Egyptian models precisely in the direction of that realism for which Greek Art is distinguished.

If we would judge how direct and unequivocal was the impulse, which the dying nation transferred to the adolescent in point of art, we have but to take a few steps in the British Museum from the Assyrian rooms to the wonderful hall that holds Lord Elgin's trophies from the desecrated Parthenon. Look, then, on the frieze of the bas-relief that bears the magic name of Phidias. If anything can reconcile us to the act that deprived Greece of her precious heirlooms, it is the fact that they have found lodgment here close beside their oriental prototypes, where half a million visitors each year may at least have an opportunity to learn the lesson that human progress is an accretion, a growth, a building on foundations; and, specifically, that Greek Art, no less than other forms of human culture, was an evolution, and not an isolated miracle.

Consequently, we cannot fully realize all of the Egypto-Asiatic influences on European civilization and progress until we imagine this work taken away and view the vacuum that would be left. Science would become bold and ragged; history would lose its charm and fascination; medicine would be barren and uninteresting; some of the brightest jewels would drop from the crown of literature, and the fairest garments would be shed from the shoulders of art.

Some of these southwestern Asiatic races, namely, the Chaldeans, Assyrians, Babylonians, Phœnicians, Hebrews and Egyptians (our neighbors on the border land) had organized civilization long before Socrates taught philosophy or before Herodotus wrote history. These antique races had literature before most nations had letters, and art while other nations knew only war and savagery. Draper quotes Cabanis as saying specifically of the Jews, that "they were our factors and bankers before we knew how to read."

With these facts in view I have come to the conclusion that the influence of Hellenic civilization, of which I am an ardent admirer, on European culture at large has been overestimated. While in the meantime the influences exerted on Greek arts and sciences by Egypto-Asiatic civilization has a tendency in certain quarters of either being underestimated or being overlooked entirely. My main object has been to make an effort to replace the honor and credit of the forces, which contributed to the development of modern culture, medicine being only an element, where it appropriately belongs.

Author Nushan H. Kassabian, M.D.

Nushan H. Kassabian was born to middle class parents in Egin, Armenia, Asia Minor on September 12, 1866, the year after President Lincoln's assassination in America. His mother Nazenie was born in 1842 in Armenia and was the niece of the Treasurer of the former Ottoman Empire. She was very devoted to her only child Nushan and encouraged him to get a good education. Nushan's father, Harotune Kassabian, was killed during the Turkish Massacres in Armenia. Nushan attended Congressional Missionary School in Harput, Turkey, where he learned to speak English. It was while teaching school that he received a letter from home saying, "Come home, you are engaged to be married." In 1891, Nushan, who was 25 years old, was betrothed to 19-year-old Margaret Nushan Jamgochian. Soon after the wedding, Nushan, seeking a better way of life for himself and his young bride, set sail for America. He then traveled from New York to Chicago where he entered Northwestern University Medical School. It was Nushan's dream to help people and cure the deadly diseases of that time.

Four years later, in June of 1896, he graduated from Northwestern University a physician and surgeon. A year later, he sent for wife Margaret who had been a witness to the horrific massacres in Armenia. In 1898, they moved to Valton, Wisconsin, where their son Armen Lincoln was born December of 1899. Nushan, wife Margaret and two-year-old son Armen moved to the Center Street home in Coopersville, Michigan. A year later, a daughter, Araxia Mariam was born to the Kassabians. On December 31, 1911, Nushan's beloved wife Margaret passed away after battling pernicious anemia for 8 months. She was 39 years old. In the fall of 1915, Dr. Kassabian moved his office form Coopersville to Detroit. He traveled back to the Center St. office every three weeks, arriving sometimes by train and at other times driving his own Maxwell which he had purchased the year before. He continued to see his Coopersville patients once every three weeks until he sold the Center St. home in the spring of 1925. He continued his practice in Detroit for the next 30 years. Much of Dr. Kassabian's life was dedicated to finding a cure for the dreaded disease tuberculosis, since one of his early patients had died from the disease. In 1913, the doctor met renowned German physician Friedrich Franz Friedman while visiting one of Friedman's clinics in New York. Dr. Kassabian continued to keep in touch with Dr. Friedman, traveling to New York and overseas to meet with him. Dr. Kassabian wrote at least five published pamphlets and is remembered as a man who spent most of his life trying to help develop cures for the diseases of that time. His tireless work in clinics and laboratories and his research and development of many therapeutic agents, including digestive aids, has aided in the advancement of many modern day medications.

After practicing medicine for over 62 years, Dr. Nushan H. Kassabian passed away on May 13, 1960 at the age of 93, less than five years after he retired. He is buried in the Coopersville cemetery, next to wife Margaret and his mother Nazenie.

Editor Chris Heimler

Chris L. Heimler was born August 30, 1982 in Grand Rapids, Michigan to Mr. Jack J. Heimler (Boyer) and Susan M. Perrin (Haisma).

Although Chris spent part of his early childhood in Marne, Michigan and Newaygo, Michigan on Hess Lake, he was mostly raised in Coopersville, MI where his Grandparents lived. From the age of 13 and on, he and his older brother Nick were raised by their grandmother Alice E. Perrin in Coopersville, MI.

In April of 1995, Chris was instrumental in organizing, supporting, and reestablishing the Coopersville Observer newspaper. The original Coopersville Observer began November 4, 1880 and continued until 1975 when competition with larger newspapers caused the editor to discontinue the efforts for a local newspaper. Chris was employed with the Observer for one year, after which owner and founder Ron Veldman sold out to Duane and Kerri Snowdin in the spring of 1996. Kerri Snowdin is the current Editor for the local newspaper. Chris continues to support and write for the Observer as it enters it tenth year in operation. Chris is most proud of this venture as it reminds him of the previous owners of his home and the forefathers of Coopersville, who also supported and wrote in the long running local newspaper. "Being a part of a newspaper people will be able to read years and years from now is something to be very proud of," says Chris.

Chris has interviewed more than 100 famous and not so famous individuals either for private research and or newspaper articles. Many of those interviews with the famous celebrities and the not so famous individuals will be featured on his site in the near future.

Today Chris works in the Public Library system in Grand Rapids, Michigan and is working closely with friend, colleague and author Craig A. Hart on several books and projects together. The two of them have many wonderful plans for the future either together or on solo projects and are proud to release them to the public and hope they help and/or entertain the readers and viewers. Chris is mostly devoted to helping make history fun for people to learn and get people more involved with historical projects and protecting our heritage. Chris also works with multiple charitable organizations that help the betterment of humankind and help make a brighter future for our children. Chris currently resides in Coopersville, Michigan with his brother Nick and beloved Grandmother Alice Perrin in their 125-year-old Folk Victorian home.

APPENDIX A

▼

"Not the Dollar Alone"
Letter to the Editor, printed in The Coopersville Observer, *1912*

EDITOR OBSERVER: The report you had in your valued paper last week in regard to my paper read before the Grand Rapids Historical Society, does not do justice to the sentiments I had expressed. So please allow me to say a word in order that I may rectify any unfavorable impression that some readers might have taken by a superficial perusal of that short report which you had taken from the Evening Press.

It was not the lure of American dollars alone that brought Armenians to America. There were politico-economic conditions that compelled the Armenians to seek the shores of free America. Under Turkish rule the Armenians were not allowed any freedom whatever. Upon the slightest pretext they were arrested and kept in their notorious dungeons without any trial or justice until they became victims of pernicious anemia or the bacillus of tuberculosis. There was no safety of life, property, or of honor. The massacre of the Armenians in the year 1894-95 was intended to give a deadly blow to a race, who, by their progressiveness and enterprise had aroused Turkish jealousy. Armenians under those conditions could not any longer endure under the rule of the "Unspeakable Turk," as Gladstone so fittingly called them. Differing from the Turks from a racial, linguistic as well as from a religious point of view and there being no signs of any improvement, my people were simply compelled to immigrate to a country where life, property and honor was respected and protected; in fact, a place where they could worship their God according to the dictates of their conscience.

There are about 40,000 Armenians in America. One-fourth of them are in the West, the rest in the East. The number of Armenians in Grand Rapids has never exceeded sixty all told. The first one to come was Stepan Kurkjian, in 1892. His son Armen, age 14, who had no knowledge of English when he first came, within six years finished his high school course and after taking a course at Ann Arbor is now the representative of the Oliver Machine Co., St. Louis, Mo., office. The majority of them are working in furniture factories. Mr. Widdicomb, who has employed a good number of them says, "They are reliable, competent and steady workmen."

Dr. N. H. Kassabian

APPENDIX B

▼

"Lectured in Grand Rapids"
printed in The Coopersville Observer, *December 4, 1908*

Dr. Kassabian gave an address on "Asiatic Civilization and Its Influence Upon European Culture" before the Ladies Literary Club in Grand Rapids one day last week in Sunday's editions of the Grand Rapids Herald. The lecture was replete with historic interest and portions of the talk were illustrated with an exhibition of oriental rugs and photographs.

The doctor confined his remarks to the historic races of southwestern Asia and paid a fine tribute to the Israelites. He said in part:-

"The Jews have been scoffed at and ridiculed, but we cannot ignore the debt we owe them. When Disraeli was attacked in parliament and scornfully called a Jew, he replied: 'Yes, I am a Jew and when the ancestors of the honorable gentleman were savages of the forest, mine were priests in the temple.' Israel matured before the world had letters. The Jews have not only given the world some of the greatest men, but also they have given the world the knowledge of the only true and living God. Jesus was a Jew and a gift of the Orient for the progress and advancement of the world.

"The influence of the Hellenic civilization upon the European culture at large has been over-estimated, while influence exerted upon Greek arts and science by Egypto-Asiatic civilization has a tendency of being either under-estimated or overlooked entirely. By and analysis of the stimulant that the Greeks received from Egypt and western Asia we will be able to replace the honor and credit upon those nations of remote antiquity, whose culture the Greeks imitated and transmitted the same to Rome and Europe. The rise and the first gems of art and architecture must be sought in the valley of the Nile and the Euphrates and not in the neighborhood of the Athenian acropolis. Plato and Solon resided for some years in Egypt in the hope of gaining an insight into the mysteries of Oriental philosophy. The Israelites were the transmitter of Chaldean religion, science and civilization to the world and thru this wonderful people their culture has become the heritage of all mankind while its science of civilization thru the medium of the Greeks and Romans have been the basis of modern research. The Babylonian culture was the oldest in the world and at the same time, the mother of all other civilizations of antiquity cannot be disputed. The study of ancient history will teach us the lessons that human progress is a growth, a building upon a foundation, and the Greco-European art, no less than other forms of human culture, was an evolution and not an isolated miracle or a new creation.

"Persia learned the fine art of rug weaving in connection with the rest of their arts and cultures from the Babylonians and Assyrians and transmitted the same to Minor Asiatic races who also in the course of time influenced the Greeks. And if we would correctly understand the development of Egypt-Mesopotamian civilization, we will readily see that our own culture is its direct outgrowth."

Glossary

Achilles Character in Greek mythology who fought in the war against Troy. *(as found on page 6)*

Aeschylus (525-456 BC) The first great tragic dramatist of Greece. *(as found on page 7)*

Aesclepiadae Descendents of Aesculapius. *(as found on pages 6 and 8)*

Aesclepion at Cos Sanatorium on the island of Cos. *(as found on page 7)*

Aesculapius Greek god of medicine. *(as found on page 6)*

Alexandria More than 2,000 years ago the capital and greatest city of Egypt. *(as found on page 7)*

Alum Potassium aluminum sulfate or an ammonium aluminum sulfate. *(as found on page 3)*

Amulets Charm designed to protect the wearer from evil. *(as found on page 4)*

Anaxagoras (5th century BC) First Western philosopher to distinguish between mind and body. *(as found on page 7)*

Anemia Condition in which the blood is deficient in red blood cells, in hemoglobin, or in total volume. *(as found on page 3)*

Aretaeus Greek physician in the 2nd century AD. *(as found on page 8)*

Ascitic fluid Serous fluid that accumulates in the abdomen. *(as found on page 8)*

Asia Minor Peninsula which lies between the Black and Mediterranean Seas and an important crossroads in ancient times. *(as found on page 1)*

Assyria War-like country of the upper Tigris Valley. *(as found on page 9)*

Assyrians Ancient, war-like people north of Babylonia. *(as found on page 1)*

Athenian acropolis Ceremonial site in Athens, Greece. *(as found on page 1)*

Ausultation Act of listening to sounds arising within organs as an aid to diagnosis and treatment. *(as found on page 8)*

Babylonia Ancient empire in the Tigris-Euphrates Valley. *(as found on page 9)*

Caelius Aurelianus North African who wrote on acute and chronic diseases in the fifth century. *(as found on page 8)*

Caesarea City on the Mediterranean coastline between Joppa and Acco. *(as found on page 8)*

Cappadocian Person from Cappadocia, an ancient inland country in Asia Minor west of Euphrates River. *(as found on page 8)*

Cassia Coarse cinnamon bark. *(as found on page 5)*

Chai Egyptian occultist and physician who practiced medicine between 5000 to 4000 BC. *(as found on page 2)*

Chaldea Equivalent of Babylonia, named for people who set up Second Babylonian Empire in the 7th century. *(as found on page 4)*

Chiron Centaur of Greek mythology who was wise in medicines. *(as found on page 6)*

Claudius Galen Most renowned physician in ancient Rome trained in Hippocratic medicine. Became imperial physician of Rome in AD 168. *(as found on page 7)*

Clysters Process used to alleviate intestinal problems. *(as found on pages 1 and 2)*

Code of Khammurabi Collection of Babylonians laws developed during the reign of Hammurabi (1792-1750 BC). *(as found on page 5)*

Constantine (AD 280?-337) First Christian emperor of Rome. *(as found on page 8)*

Constantinople City on the Black Sea that Emperor Constantine made his capital in AD 330. *(as found on page 8)*

Corinth City in a small state in south central part of ancient Greece. *(as found on page 7)*

Demosthenes (384-322 BC) Greatest of the Greek orators. *(as found on page 7)*

Diodorus (died about 20 BC) Greek historian of time of Julius Caesar and Augustus. *(as found on page 9)*

Draughts Portion poured out or mixed for drinking. *(as found on page 3)*

Embalming Using preservatives to maintain a dead body as long as possible. *(as found on page 2)*

Emetics Causing to vomit. *(as found on page 2)*

Empyema Condition in which pus fills the spaces surrounding the lungs. *(as found on page 8)*

Etiology All of the causes of a disease or abnormal condition, a branch of knowledge dealing with causes. *(as found on page 7)*

Euphrates Longest river in western Asia at 1,700 miles. *(as found on page 1)*

Eurypides (484?-406 BC) The third of the great Greek tragic poets. *(as found on page 7)*

Fellows, Sir Charles (1799-1860) British archaeologist. Discovered fourteen old Greek cities in Turkey. *(as found on page 9)*

Hadrian (AD 76-138) Publius Aelius Hadrianus, called Hadrian, was Roman emperor from AD 117 until 138. *(as found on page 7)*

Helena Mother of the Emperor Constantine. *(as found on page 8)*

Heliopolis Ancient Egyptian city, once the seat of sun worship. *(as found on page 2)*

Hellas Originally a small district of Thessaly, later signifying all of ancient Greece. *(as found on page 5)*

Hellenic race Greeks. *(as found on page 1)*

Hematuria Presence of blood or blood cells in the urine. *(as found on page 3)*

Heraclides Greek philosopher of the fourth century AD. *(as found on page 6)*

Herodotus (484?-425? BC) "Father of History" and one of the most widely traveled people of his time. *(as found on pages 5, 7, 8 and 10)*

Hieroglyphics Ancient Egyptian system of writing. *(as found on page 2)*

Hippocrates "Father of Medicine", first name in the history of medicine. *(as found on page 6)*

Homer Ancient Greek poet who lived around 850 BC. *(as found on page 6)*

Ionic column Form of architecture characterized by especially by the spiral volutes of its capital. *(as found on page 9)*

Island of Cos Island in ancient Greece and home of Hippocrates. *(as found on page 6)*

Jerusalem City in Israel which is considered a holy city by three of the world's major religions. *(as found on page 8)*

Judea Greek and Roman name for south Palestine. *(as found on page 5)*

Laennec (1781-1826). Laennec, Rene-Theophile-Hyacinthe. Considered the father of chest medicine, a French physician who invented the stethoscope. *(as found on page 8)*

Layard in Nineveh (1817-94) Layard, Austen Henry. A British archaeologist who excavated the city of Nineveh. *(as found on pages 1 and 10)*

Lord Elgin British ambassador to Turkey. *(as found on page 10)*

Lysias (459-380 BC). One of great Attic orators. *(as found on page 7)*

Macedonia Region of southeast Europe. *(as found on page 7)*

Marcus Aurelius (AD 121-180). Became the Roman emperor in AD 161. *(as found on page 7)*

Medicaments Substances used in therapy. *(as found on page 3)*

Memphis Early capital of Egypt now in ruins. *(as found on page 2)*

Memphite stone Substance used in Egyptian medicine which, when mixed with certain chemicals could inhibit pain. *(as found on page 3)*

Mesopotamia Area between the Tigris and Euphrates rivers in what is now Iraq. *(as found on page 9)*

Miltiades (died 488? BC) Athenian general who won victory over the Persians at Marathon. *(as found on page 7)*

Milton (1608-74) Milton, John. One of the greatest English poets and author of "Paradise Lost". *(as found on page 1)*

Moses Leader of the Israelites during the Exodus from Egypt. *(as found on page 6)*

Mucilaginous Being moist and viscid or secreting mucilage. *(as found on page 3)*

Nebsu Egyptian physician who practiced medicine between 5000 to 4000 BC. *(as found on page 2)*

Necromancers One who practices the conjuring of spirits of the dead for purposes of magically revealing the future or influencing the course of events. *(as found on page 4)*

Nicias (died 413 BC) Athenian statesman and general in the Peloponnesian War. *(as found on page 7)*

Nile River in Africa and the longest in the world at 4,132 miles. *(as found on page 1)*

Niter Potassium or sodium nitrate. *(as found on page 3)*

Obstetrics Branch of medical science that deals with birth and with its antecedents and sequels. *(as found on page 7)*

Ophthalmia Inflammation of the conjunctiva or eyeball. *(as found on page 2)*

Osiris Egyptian god of sun, health and agriculture. *(as found on page 2)*

Palestine Region between the Jordan River and the Mediterranean Sea. *(as found on page 7)*

Patroclus In Greek mythology, hero of the Trojan War and friend of Achilles. *(as found on page 6)*

Paul of Aegina Greek physician who worked in the seventh? century. Wrote a seven volume medical history. *(as found on page 8)*

Percussion Act or technique of tapping of tapping the surface of a body part to learn the condition of the parts beneath by the resultant sound. *(as found on page 8)*

Perdicas King of Macedonia who was treated and healed by Hippocrates. *(as found on page 7)*

Pergamus (Pergamum) Celebrated ancient city of north west Asia Minor. *(as found on page 7)*

Pericles (495?-429? BC) Statesman who opened Athenian democracy to the ordinary citizen. *(as found on page 7)*

Persepolis Ancient capital of the Persian Empire. *(as found on page 9)*

Persia Land between the Caspian Sea and the Persian Gulf. *(as found on page 6)*

Persian Wars Attempt by the vast Persian Empire in the 5th century BC to conquer Greece. *(as found on page 8)*

Phidias (490?-430? BC). Athenian sculptor who directed the building of the Parthenon. *(as found on page 10)*

Phoenicia Land of the Phoenicians located on the Syrian coast. *(as found on page 6)*

Phoenicians Skillful mariners of ancient times. *(as found on page 1)*

Phthisis Pulmonary tuberculosis. *(as found on page 8)*

Plato (428?-348? BC) Greek philosopher. The most celebrated teacher of his day. *(as found on pages 2 and 7)*

Polytheistic religion Belief or worship of many gods. *(as found on page 1)*

Pythagoras (580?-500? BC) Greek philosopher and mathematician who was instrumental in formulating principles which influenced Plato and Aristotle. *(as found on page 7)*

Pythagoreans Group of people who believed reality, at its deepest level, is mathematical in nature. *(as found on page 2)*

Sakhit Egyptian god who treated bone fractures by the intercession of the goddess. *(as found on page 2)*

Schlegel (1772-1829) Schlegel, Karl Wilhelm Friedrich von. German critic, scholar and poet. *(as found on page 2)*

Scythia Name applied by ancient Greeks to the steppes north of the Black Sea. *(as found on page 7)*

Socrates (470?-399?) Greek philosopher and considered the wisest of his time. *(as found on page 7)*

Solon (630?-560? BC). Greek statesman and poet. *(as found on page 8)*

Soothsayers One who practices the foretelling of events. *(as found on page 4)*

Sophocles (496?-406 BC) The second of the three great Greek writers of tragic drama. *(as found on page 7)*

Soronnes of Ephesus Physician who practiced in Rome during the time of Trajan and Hadrian, from 98 to 138 AD. *(as found on page 7)*

Sprengel, Kurt (1766-1833) German botanist and physician born in Pomerania. *(as found on page 1)*

Sputum Expectorated matter made up of saliva and often discharged from the respiratory passages. *(as found on page 8)*

Succussion Action or process of shaking or the state of being shaken, especially with violence. *(as found on page 8)*

Talisman Something producing apparently magical or miraculous effects. *(as found on page 4)*

Teta Egyptian king and physician who practiced medicine between 5000 to 4000 BC. *(as found on page 2)*

Thebes Capital of ancient Egypt at the height of its' power. *(as found on page 2)*

Themistocles (524?-460? BC) Creator of the Athenian navy during the wars of the Greeks against the Persians. *(as found on page 7)*

Thessaly Region in Greece south of Macedonia. *(as found on page 7)*

Thucydides (460?-404?) Great Athenian historian. *(as found on page 7)*

Trajan (AD 53?-117) Trajanus, Marcus Ulpius. Roman emperor 98-117. *(as found on page 7)*

Tsethosta Egyptian king and physician who practiced medicine between 5000 to 4000 BC. *(as found on page 2)*

Tympanites Distension of the abdomen caused by accumlumation of gas in the intestinal tract or peritoneal cavity. *(as found on page 8)*

Ulysses (Odysseus) In Greek mythology, king of Ithaca and Trojan War hero. *(as found on page 6)*

Ur of the Chaldeas Ancient city of south Babylonia near the Euphrates River. *(as found on page 9)*

Xenophon (430?-355? BC). The Greek historian who wrote of the military campaigns in which he served as a young officer. *(as found on page 7)*

Zantian marbles Zantian products composed or made of marble, particularly sculptures. *(as found on page 9)*

Bibliography[1]

1. "Sprengel, Kurt." *The 1911 Edition Encyclopedia.* Online. PageWise, Inc. 1911. www.1911ency.org. (10/11/02).

2. "Herbal Preparations: Enemas/Clysters." *Tempest Wolf's Lair.* Online. 2002. http://www.tempestwolf.com/herbs/herbs/herbalprep/enemas.htm. (10/11/02).

3. "acropolis." *Encyclopedia.com.* Online. 2002. http://www.encyclopedia.com/html/a1/acropoli.asp. (10/11/02).

4. Arab, Sameh M., MD. "Medicine in Ancient Egypt; Part 2 of 3." *Arab World Books.* Online. http://www.arabworldbooks.com/articles8b.htm. (10/11/02).

5. *Compton's Interactive Encyclopedia.* 2000 ed. CD-ROM. Cambridge, MA: The Learning Company, 1999.

6. *Webster's Seventh New Collegiate Dictionary.* Springfield, Mass: G. & C. Merriam Company, 1963.

7. Laney, J. Carl. *Concise Bible Atlas.* 2nd Edition ed. Peabody: Hendrickson Publishers, Inc., 1999.

---

1. These sources were used mainly to compile the preceding glossary. Unfortunately, most sources used in the writing of the actual piece were unavailable, as they were not listed by the original author. If a specific source is recognized, please feel free to contact the editor and we will do what we can to include it in any subsequent editions.

8. "Paul of Aegina." *Bartleby.com*. Online. 2001. http://www.bartleby.com/65/pa/PaulAegi.html. (10/12/02).

9. "History of Medicine Review." *Voyageur*. Online. 2000. http://www.voyageur.drake.edu/Bio_198/hist_med_rev_2.html. (10/12/02).

10. "Sir Charles Fellows." *Find A Grave*. Online. 1999. http://www.findagrave.com/cgi-bin/fg.cgi?page=gr&GRid=6583. (10/12/02).

Armenian Resources on the Web

Armenian Youth Federation: http://www.ayf.org/
Armenia Fund: http://www.armeniafund.org/
Armenian Genocide: http://www.genocide1915.info/
Government of Republic of Armenia:
http://www.gov.am/enversion/index.html
Asbarez Armenian Daily Newspaper: http://www.asbarez.com/
Armenian News Agency: http://www.armenpress.am/

Index

0-595-33501-2

www.ingramcontent.com/pod-product-compliance
Lightning Source LLC
Chambersburg PA
CBHW021042180526
45163CB00005B/2251